Administration of a
Radiology Department

ADMINISTRATION OF A
RADIOLOGY DEPARTMENT

Hints for Day-to-Day Operation

By

MURRAY L. JANOWER, M.D.

Physician-in-Chief, Department of Radiology
The St. Vincent Hospital
Worcester, Massachusetts
Associate Professor of Radiology
University of Massachusetts Medical School
Clinical Associate in Radiology
Massachusetts General Hospital
Lecturer in Radiology
Harvard Medical School
Boston, Massachusetts

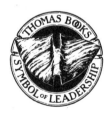

CHARLES C THOMAS • **PUBLISHER**
Springfield • *Illinois* • *U.S.A.*

Published and Distributed Throughout the World by
CHARLES C THOMAS • PUBLISHER
Bannerstone House
301-327 East Lawrence Avenue, Springfield, Illinois, U.S.A.

© *1976, by* CHARLES C THOMAS • PUBLISHER

ISBN 0-398-03514-8

Library of Congress Catalog Card Number: 75-35567

With THOMAS BOOKS *careful attention is given to all details of manufacturing and design. It is the Publisher's desire to present books that are satisfactory as to their physical qualities and artistic possibilities and appropriate for their particular use.* THOMAS BOOKS *will be true to those laws of quality that assure a good name and good will.*

Printed in the United States of America
R-1

Library of Congress Cataloging in Publication Data

Janower, Murray L
     Administration of a radiology department.

     1. Hospitals--Radiological services--Administra-
tion. I. Title. [DNLM: 1. Hospital departments.
2. Hospital administration. 3. Radiology. WX221
J34a]
RA975.5.R3J36   658'.91'36210425   75-35567
ISBN 0-398-03514-8

To Linda, Julie, Amy and Andrew

PREFACE

THE purpose of this book is to demonstrate that the application of common sense and sound business management principles to a radiology department will result in a marked improvement in its day-to-day operation. The book is not intended to be an exhaustive treatment, and the suggested methodology is not necessarily the best. The systems described in the following pages work in one specific department; but all departments are different, and what works in one environment might be totally inappropriate in another. The systems were originally developed in one of the diagnostic radiology divisions at the Massachusetts General Hospital where 125,000 examinations per year were performed; they were then modified at St. Vincent Hospital, Worcester, Massachusetts, where the annual volume is 75,000 examinations.

The basis of this book is the refresher course that I have given for a number of years at the annual meeting of The Radiological Society of North America. Many people have expressed an interest in this subject and have requested printed material. I have expanded my notes greatly and have added many facts and figures not previously presented.

ACKNOWLEDGMENTS

THIS book and these ideas would not have been possible without the help of many people.

Of these, I must first acknowledge Mr. Charles Bianchi, R.T., my department administrator, who is both my right- and left-hand man. Dr. Stephen Balter, radiation physicist, helped in the development of many of these ideas. My dear colleagues Doctors Karl Benedict, Jr., Peter Chen, and Milton Weiner have had to put up with many different experiments in their daily practice of radiology and have held up surprisingly well. Mrs. Suzanne Caldwell, my secretary, has retyped the drafts of these notes so many times that she knows them by heart.

Finally, the medical staff and the hospital administration (David Hannan, in particular) at St. Vincent Hospital have been most supportive.

M.L.J.

CONTENTS

Administration of a
Radiology Department

CHAPTER 1

--- --- --- --- --- --- --- --- --- --- --- --- --- --- --- --- --- --- --- ---

INTRODUCTION

--- --- --- --- --- --- --- --- --- --- --- --- --- --- --- --- --- --- --- ---

THE diagnostic radiologist is one of the most skilled superspecialists in the medical field, possessing expertise in most areas of medical practice. His skills are used in the care of most hospitalized patients, and he contributes to the medical well-being of over 100,000,000 Americans who undergo radiological examinations each year. Yet, something is lacking. It is not uncommon to find radiological departments resembling huge battlefields with long lines of patients, unbelievable amounts of noise, dozens of confused personnel, angry clinicians, and harassed radiologists. Why is it that the radiologist is capable of saving a human life but may be unable to find film envelopes on large numbers of patients? Is it possible that a superspecialist who contributes so much to the education and organization of medical students' minds is unable to organize his own department to insure that there is not a three-day delay from the time he dictates a report until it reaches the clinician? Can it be possible that the radiologist is lacking in knowledge or is unwilling to make the effort to correct the chaotic circumstances in which he works? As a practicing radiologist, the author must answer the above questions with an emphatic "no."

The radiologist's problems stems from his lack of management skills. This is not surprising since there is usually no time devoted to this subject in medical schools or resident training programs. It is the purpose of this book to analyze the functions of a radiology department in a way that will be applicable to each radiologist's individual practice situation.

It will be useful to mention a few basic management principles which must be enforced. The most important of these are *planning* and *analysis*. These are processes in which the individuals concerned in a department's operations meet and develop methods for performing their functions as efficiently as possible. The planning process must involve the people doing the work, as they are the ones who best understand their jobs. Furthermore, it is gratifying to the workers to participate in the planning and analysis processes and easier for them to implement plans that they have helped develop.

The next management objectives are *leading* and *delegating*. The chief must be available to everyone within the department, but it is impossible for him to oversee every detail. Most chiefs of radiology departments are unable to delegate authority; they feel that they must participate in every decision, however small. When authority is properly delegated, most of the minor decisions, and many of the major ones, are made by the people most intimately associated with the problem, namely the people performing the tasks. Delegation must be clearly designated, and the involved individuals must be given reasonable autonomy.

Delegation of authority has many important benefits. Assigning authority to different people greatly increases their motivation. It also brings increased numbers of people into the decision-making process. Although the ultimate authority still rests with the chief, the additional opinions brought to bear on the subject are valuable.

An excellent example of the delegation process can be seen in the role of the administrative assistant within the department. Most departments of reasonable size must have a full-time administrative assistant who should be distinguished from the chief technologist; the chief technologist is primarily concerned with patient care in the department on a practical level. The title administrative assistant is a poor one; the person in this job should properly be called the radiology department administrator (RDA). The chief must have complete trust in the RDA, and he must permit the RDA to function on a semiautonomous basis.

The job protocol for the RDA is shown in Figure 1. The RDA is in charge of the day-to-day running of the department; he can make at least 90 percent of the necessary decisions. Chiefs who have difficulty delegating authority may hold weekly or even daily briefing conferences with the RDA. For example, many chiefs of departments see all detail men who come to their departments; but the RDA could easily meet with these individuals to form a preliminary opinion on new products. The RDA could then summarize his opinions for the chief, saving him substantial amounts of time. The chief may reserve authority to make final decisions on new products, and may overrule the RDA's opinion if they disagree; this almost never happens in the author's department.

Figure 1

JOB DESCRIPTION

RADIOLOGY DEPARTMENT ADMINISTRATOR

SUMMARY
Is responsible on a daily basis for all administrative and technical services associated with the routine planning and operation of radiology services.
RESPONSIBLE TO:
Chief of Radiology
WORK PERFORMED
    I. Planning with the chief for
        A. Department manpower requirements
        B. Equipment needs
        C. Operating supplies
    II. Budgeting annually with the chief for the needs of the department.
    III. Supervising on a routine daily basis
        A. Technician education
        B. Quality of the work accomplished in the department
        C. Clerical support functions associated with operations
        D. Technical and repair services
    IV. Controlling on a routine and daily basis
        A. Departmental systems and operations
        B. Departmental expenses through the use of budgetary guidelines
    V. Coordinating routine daily operations and planning with other Hospital departments.
ACCOUNTABLE FOR
    I. Satisfactory routine daily operation of radiology department.
    II. Accuracy and productivity of personnel supervised.
    III. Accuracy and productivity of work performed.
    IV. Objective appraisal of the performance of personnel supervised.
    V. Periodic evaluation of equipment to insure continued top performance.
    VI. The proper expenditure of financial resources as fixed by budget guidelines.

Qualifications
  I.   Appropriate registrations
  II. Five years' experience as chief technol-
       ogist
  III. Three years of pertinent top management
       and planning experience in radiology de-
       partment

In addition to the basic principles outlined above, there are a few mandatory rules which must be applied to the department. Taken together, they typify a state of mind. Without this state of mind, running a department smoothly is impossible. The application of these rules will be demonstrated repeatedly in subsequent chapters.

The first of these is the clear identification of major categories of functions within a department. This is followed by a detailed analysis of steps involved in fulfilling those functions including the development of a written protocol by the individuals working in the area. The protocol should result in a step-by-step how-to manual which must answer the standard questions of who, what, when, why, how, and where. A stranger walking into the work area should be able to perform the job (albeit with difficulty) by following this step-by-step outline.

For example, if one were considering film handling, there would be a minimum of nine major functions that would be initially identified (Fig. 2); subsequently, each of these functions would be delineated on a step-by-step basis including the individual responsible. The development of these written protocols is a difficult, time-consuming, frustrating task, but the rewards more than compensate for the effort involved.

Figure 2

SEQUENCE OF FILM HANDLING

1. File clerk gets old film retrieval information.
2. Old jacket retrieved.
3. Old jacket put in temporary file.
4. New films are delivered from darkroom to
   file room.

```
5.  New films are collated with old films.
6.  All films delivered to reading room.
7.  Films are interpreted.
8.  Films are returned to file room.
9.  Films are placed in master files.
```

Once each protocol has been developed, it must be integrated with the work protocols from other areas in the department. Overlaps will be encountered which are usually readily corrected; functions are then assigned to specific individuals. An important part of this principle is the stress placed on having jobs performed by a person at his or her proper level of training. For example, a messenger cannot function as a registered technologist, and a technologist should not function as a messenger. We call the process of dividing complex tasks into their basic elements and assigning of specific individuals to each task, the Partition-Responsibility Principle. Running an efficient department hinges on this principle.

The first step in departmental analysis is the identification of the major functioning units. It is useful to think of these units in the order that a patient must follow when obtaining a radiological examination. They are as follows:

1. Patient scheduling and control
2. Performance of the examination
3. Filing
4. Interpretation of the examination
5. Transcription of the report

Each of these subdivisions is an important entity within the department. If something goes wrong in any one of these areas, the entire operation can be upset.

Once the major units have been identified, written flow sheets for each of these operations must be developed by the people involved in each of the operations. As the protocol is developed, immediate inefficiencies will become apparent. For example, the fact that films can be found in the file room is apparent. What must be spelled out is how the films are found and who is doing the finding.

The application of the Partition-Responsibility Principle can be shown in one large diagnostic department which is divided into chest, bone, GI, GU, and subspecialties. These major divisions are subdivided into operational subunits as shown in Figures 3 and 4. In charge of each subdivision is a radiologist. This individual now has increased responsibilities. Beneath him are several junior staff radiologists, some of whom are permanently assigned to the division, while others rotate on a monthly basis. In charge of each area is a technologist who also has come permanent and rotational junior technologists beneath him or her. Each subspecialty has its own secretary and file room clerks assigned to it. In other words, each subspecialty is a complete unit and yet belongs to a whole. Each subclassification of employee also reports laterally to the paramedical person in charge of similar personnel within the department. For example, all secretaries report to the chief secretary and all technologists to the chief technologist. The prime responsibility of the secretary and the technologist in each section is, however, to the radiologist in charge of that section.

The result of the assignment of responsibility should be self-evident. When the gastrointestinal fluoroscopy reports are not being transcribed promptly there is one specific secretary who can be singled out from the secretarial pool. When the GI films are not being assembled promptly for interpretation, there is one person in the file room who is having difficulty in fulfilling his job. It should be noted that the inability of certain people to fulfill their job function does not mean that these individuals are not making a maximum effort. There may be problems in the system which prohibit them from functioning properly. However, they are in an excellent position to identify these problems and the problems can then usually be corrected quickly.

In this book, a description of a department performing 75,000 annual examinations is given. It is run on a modified appointment basis where all patients are called to the floor from one central point. Radiological technologists take x-ray films, which is what they are trained to do, and perform few other functions which can be performed by people with lesser training. Film interpretation is done using a multiple view box system, with specific people assigned to specific tasks. The overall work en-

MAJOR DIVISIONS WITHIN A DEPARTMENT

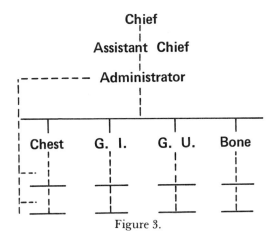

Figure 3.

SUBUNITS WITHIN A MAJOR DIVISION

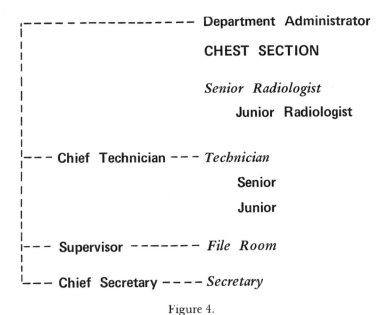

Figure 4.

vironment is pleasant and peaceful. Patients are treated with dignity with an average stay in the department of less than forty minutes. Films of excellent quality are obtained and few of these films are lost. Most of the reports of these examinations are in the patient's chart by that evening.

CHAPTER 2

PATIENT CONTROL

THE goal of the radiology department is to perform the needed number of x-ray examinations in a maximally efficient manner with all rooms used to their capacity and minimum patient waiting periods. This is a yeoman's task, as the department has no control over its input. Workloads within the department may vary by as much as 25 to 50 percent from day to day, and planning must be done on the maximum workload, not the average.

This chapter is concerned with the method in which patients are brought to the radiology department, handled while on the floor, and returned to their points of origin. There are many different systems in use. In one common system, a number of requisitions are delivered in the morning to the different technologists in different rooms, who then have the responsibility for calling patients to the floor. This method guarantees that the technologist will spend more time using the telephone than the x-ray machine. In addition, there may be times in the day when all rooms call patients simultaneously. Obviously, there are not enough messengers to deliver these patients to the rooms at the same time. Even if there were enough messengers, ten new patients entering the department simultaneously would create a traffic jam. Furthermore, it is difficult to know which patients have already been to the department or are in the department at a given time.

Another system, and perhaps the one most frequently encountered, consists of placing all requisitions in one large pile, beginning to call patients at the top of the pile, and racing throughout the day hoping to reach the bottom of the pile by nightfall. This system is to be condemned.

In an efficient system, all patients should be called to the de-

11

partment from one central point; 200 patients can be handled in this fashion, using a manual system, by 1½ people per day. These persons, called control officers, should preferably be x-ray technologists, although it is not mandatory. This would be an excellent place for computer application, and it may be that the computer may make the job somewhat easier. However, it will be some time before most hospitals can afford computers; furthermore, one will still have the individual-computer interface to deal with. The individual controlling the computer, rather than the presence of the computer, is the key factor in the smooth operation of the department.

The control officer works closely with the receptionist. For a department seeing 200 patients per day, two receptionists are required. Accordingly, 3½ to 4 people are required to meet the patients as they come to the floor and to arrange for the patients to arrive at and leave the floor. The receptionist also answers all telephone calls made to the department; in a large department there may be over 100 calls per day.

A problem that is frequently encountered in radiology departments is the patient index system, and there are many systems in use in this country. A common system is the assignment of a different x-ray number to the patient each time he comes to the department. The extreme difficulty of integrating this number with previous numbers and the integration of new films with previous examinations should be obvious.

If a separate x-ray number from the main hospital patient number must be used, this number should be assigned to the patient the first time he comes to the radiology department, and should remain as the patient's number at all subsequent visits. The most common system of maintaining the patient index is the use of a role-type file in which individual index cards are alphabetically placed. Given trays can be obtained by pressing an appropriate button which indicates a certain section of the alphabet. This system is bulky and inefficient. As the number of patients increases, the number of cards becomes difficult to handle, and overcrowding is a common situation. Errors within such a system will average a minimum of 15 percent.

The recent advances in microfilm and microfiche offer a solution to this problem. A typical fiche measures four by five inches and one fiche can hold identifying information on up to 2000 patients. A given name can be found in less than fifteen seconds. The difficulties in using microfilm have also been overcome with the development of a new generation of microfilm readers. Whether a fiche or a film system is used will depend upon what is available in the geographical area.

If one decides to convert to a miniature system, it must be decided whether the whole index system (both old and new patients) should be converted initially, or whether the new system will be used only with new patients, while the old system slowly ages itself out of existence. The former alternative is vastly preferable. The method of conversion of the old cards to the fiche or film system will again depend on the capability of service bureaus in one's area. In one case, each of the 100,000 cards was keypunched for computer preparation of the microfiche. To accomplish this objective a personnel agency supplied 2000 work-hours at $3.00 per hour over a three-month period. To correct the errors transmitted from the old card file took an additional 480 work-hours. Punch cards were had at a total cost of approximately $7400 from which the computer generated microfiches. Data included patient name, number, address, birth date, sex, and date of last examination. It was not necessary to list all previous examinations as these could easily be found on the master film folder.

Once the fiche or film is put into use, a method of updating it must be developed. One method is to prepare a new set of fiche once a month. Between updating, current examinations can be kept in a manual card file. In a department performing 75,000 examinations annually, one will find approximately 200 cards at the end of the first day after the new fiche arrive and 4000 cards by the end of the month. It can, therefore, be seen that, although some cards are still used in this system, their numbers have been drastically reduced. This updating function costs $200 per month plus another $200 per month for rental of fiche readers. While these costs are substantial, it is axiomatic that the first step in serving a patient in the department is his proper identification.

The ideal situation is found in those hospitals in which a hospital wide unit-number system is used. Under this system, the patient is assigned a permanent number when he enters the hospital, and this number is used in all departments. It has been suggested by some that the social security number be used as this unique identifying number. In these days of concern over personal freedom, many are reluctant to do this for fear that the social security number might be abused.

The system presented below is essentially a modified appointment scheme. Basic to this scheme is the fact that all patients are scheduled for their examinations; no patients may be sent to the department without prior notification and approval of the department. For inpatients other than emergencies, all requests for examinations must be in the department by 4 P.M. of the previous day. (In actuality, we accept requisitions until 8 A.M. of that day.) It is not infrequent in large hospitals for the outpatient department, clinics, and emergency room to send patients to the radiology department at any time they feel it necessary. Obviously, if ten patients enter the department simultaneously from the busy clinics, it may be several hours until that tenth patient can be accommodated. In the system under discussion, the clinics call the department before sending patients over, and they are then given the earliest possible appointment. This may be immediately, or there may be a delay of several hours. During this time the patient is able to have lunch, have a coffee break, or go for a walk. When the patient arrives in the department, he must be taken immediately, and with careful planning this is usually possible. The patients are much happier under this system and so is the radiology department.

In order to schedule patients, one must have some idea as to which examinations will be done in what rooms, and each room should have a specific function. The most obvious, mandatory in most departments, is the room where all chest examinations are performed. If a patient comes to the department requiring several examinations, including a chest film, he will have to be handled in more than one room. While some departments may require an automated chest unit in which the films are automatically fed into the processor, there are many departments which can get along with more simple equipment. For example, an x-ray tube coupled to a wall bucky grid with a phototimer is one method by which excellent chest films can be obtained. Some radiologists resist the thought of having a single room devoted to chest examinations because they feel that the room will not be occupied completely during the day. However, it must be noted that in most departments a minimum of 40 percent of the workload is chests. If it is possible to handle almost one half of all patients entering the department in one room, thus freeing all other rooms for the other patients, it is to everyone's advantage.

The number of fluoroscopic examinations which can be performed is related to the number of fluoroscopic rooms. If each fluoroscopic patient requires twenty minutes in a room, this means that each room should handle three patients per hour. Indeed, this does not sound as if the room is very busy. However, if fluoroscopy is done from 8 A.M. until noon, and three patients per hour are examined in each of three rooms, thirty-six fluoroscopic examinations can easily be performed during a morning.

Another area which lends itself to scheduling is intravenous urography. If one allows one hour per patient, and if there are two rooms devoted to intravenous urograms, sixteen examinations per day can be performed. For those patients that are going to be examined in the afternoon, the floors are notified and the patients are permitted a light breakfast.

There is one other system which may be preferential for performance of intravenous urograms; that is, to have a patient in every room in the department at 7 A.M., have the patient injected promptly, and have the examination over at 8 A.M. In a ten-room department, this means that by 8 A.M., ten intravenous urograms would be completed. Unfortunately, it is difficult to arrange to have enough messengers, technologists, or radiologists present to have this system function properly.

Having accounted for the chest examinations, fluoroscopies, and intravenous urograms, approximately 30 percent of the workload, consisting primarily of bone work, is left. In general, fifteen minutes is allowed for each of these other examinations, although a patient requiring multiple bone examinations may require up to one hour per room. It should be noted that the fluoroscopy rooms are available in the afternoon for routine work. In one ten-room department, rooms are divided as follows:

fluoroscopy — 3; IVP — 2; chest — 1, specials — 1; other — 3.

The Partition-Responsibility Theory and the division of labor into the smallest possible units is well demonstrated here. This analysis of room utilization is much simpler and more straightforward than it would be if considered in other large units, such as the more convential division of a certain number of square feet per patient.

The above comments on the number of rooms required to perform a certain number of examinations are based on the assumption that standard cassettes are used in which films must be manually fed into a processor. However, a new generation of equipment which encompasses automatic collimation, phototiming, and automatic loading of the x-ray machine and processor is rapidly becoming available. With a vertical unit used for chest films and a horizontal unit used for table work (bucky films), it will be possible to perform approximately 75 percent of a daily workload of 200 cases in two rooms. The space requirements for departments will be markedly reduced in the near future.

Scheduling can be accomplished on either a time or a daily basis. Schemes are available whereby workloads are distributed during the day by time. The distribution of patients by room and time can be done by the technologist working the midnight shift, who will know of at least 60 percent of the examinations for the following day. As the technologist distributes patients by room and time, he keeps in mind the fact that there will be a number of unannounced outpatient and emergency room patients as well as inpatient emergencies that require examinations during the following day. Gaps can then be left within the schedule which will be filled in by these categories of patients. The inpatients can be given relatively firm time commitments, leaving time slots which are filled in by the unannounced and emergency patients. Time scheduling done by the hour is usually adequate for most departments.

It may be easier to schedule patients by room and day leaving greater flexibility in time. The nighttime technologist distributes patients by room determined by the type of examination; obviously, the patient who is first on the list will be called first during the day and the patient who is last on the list will be called towards the end of the day. For example, all diabetic and pediatric patients are done early in the morning. The technologist can also deliver a schedule to each patient floor so that the nurses have some idea as to the time of day that their patients will be called to the radiology department. When the workday begins, the control officer is presented with a schedule. We have used a two by three foot chart on which each radiographic room is assigned its own column (Fig. 5). Under each section is a place for the patient's name and room number, and the times at which the patient arrives on the floor, goes into the room, comes out of the room, and is discharged from the department.

REPRESENTATIVE EXAMPLES FROM THE CONTROL SHEET

	CHEST ROOM					FLUOROSCOPY ROOM I			
Name	Time Arrive	In	Out	Discharge	Name	Time Arrive	In	Out	Discharge

Figure 5.

The control officer first alerts the floor that a messenger will be up to collect the patient in fifteen minutes. This allows time for the patient to be properly prepared to come to the department and also lets the radiology department know if a patient is not available. A messenger is then dispatched to deliver the patient to the appropriate radiographic room, and the control officer is notified when this occurs. As the patient is taken into the room, the control officer is notified by the technologist who also notifies "control" as soon as the patient leaves the room. As soon as the quality of the film has been passed, the patient is discharged from the floor by the control officer and the time is again noted.

The flow of patients to the radiology department, their length of stay on the floor, and their dismissal from the department is, therefore, controlled by a central point. A fine thermostat is at work consisting of communication among the technologists, film quality control, the messengers, and the control officer. The technologists in their rooms alert the control officer as to their needs. If an examination which should be rapidly performed turns into an unmitigated mess, this fact is relayed to the control officer. The control officer also has his own feeling for the needs of the room. For example, he or she knows that if a patient has been called for an abdominal examination in a room, another patient must be ready for that room within a ten-minute period. If there is difficulty in a room, the control officer is notified by the technologist and delays calling another patient for that room. The thermostat places the direct responsibility for operating efficiency of a room with the technologist in that room. At the same time the technologist is relieved of the function of having to act as a telephone operator and worrying about having his or her next patient available; that is now the responsibility of the control officer.

The recorded times are primarily used to follow the patient's course through the department. If a time lapse of fifteen minutes occurs between any of the times recorded, the control officer automatically knows that some difficulty has occurred. The problem is usually that someone has forgotten about the patient. When this occurs, the control officer can identify the problem immediately and see to it that it is corrected.

The figures have other uses; if one wants to know whether or at what time a patient has been examined that day, one only has to check with the control officer. If the patient has not yet been examined, control can indicate the approximate time the patient will be called to the radiology department.

The times are also extremely valuable from the analytic point of view. The length of stay on the floor for each patient can easily be determined, and one can also decide how efficiently each room is being used. For example, it is usually readily apparent if the waiting time is too great before the examination is performed. Correspondingly, one can easily determine the time that is required for film processing; if there is difficulty in this area it should be readily apparent. The figures have further usefulness in documenting the efficiency or lack of efficiency of the department. A not infrequent occurrence is for the clinical services to raise questions as to the total duration of time the patient has spent in the radiology department. Figures are readily available in the department which substantiate or refute these claims.

This system is not perfect and it does not work all of the time. However, it is unusual in a well-run department to find long lines of patients. The goal should be to have one patient in each room and one patient waiting for each room. Accordingly, the halls may frequently look relatively barren, although the department is working at maximum efficiency.

The basic principles covered in this chapter are as follows:
1. Patients must be assigned a permanent x-ray number, preferably by a unit numbering system in use throughout the entire hospital.
2. Radiographic rooms within a department must be subspecialized by type of examination. A chest room is mandatory in most departments.
3. A modified appointment system must exist in which examinations are scheduled by room and time.
4. Patients must be called to the floor and monitored while on the floor by a central control office.

CHAPTER 3

MESSENGERS

THE transportation of patients to and from the department of radiology is frequently an area of difficulty which can easily be solvsd by the assignment of messengers to the radiology department. Most hospitals frequently have a central messenger service, and some are loath to fragment that service by assigning a few messengers to work only in radiology. However, the radiology department has greater control over several messengers assigned to it rather than to the central hospital service. Besides, this is mandated by the Partition-Responsibility Theory. Furthermore, the messengers assigned to the department feel that they belong and they have a new pride in seeing that the radiology department is properly represented. It should be remembered that the messengers are frequently the first individuals that the hospital inpatient meets from the radiology department, and the messengers should act as ambassadors of good will for the department.

Since the messenger service is frequently at the bottom of the list of job categories, the individuals who fill these jobs are also frequently near the bottom of the job skill pool. However, this does not mean that the messengers are lesser individuals or are people without skills. The messenger job, if done properly, does require certain skills including diplomacy and is a challenge to many individuals.

One department worked with both young boys from the ghetto, who essentially had never held jobs before, and with older women. The young boys originally came from the hospital pool. They appeared somewhat disinterested and lacked a clear understanding of the basic essentials of any job, i.e. that one has an assigned responsibility and should fulfill these responsibilities as a matter of individual pride, rather than secondary to supervision by a policeman. The importance of the individual's work was carefully explained to each of them and over a period of a week or so, pride in the radiology department was instilled. As the new messengers came to realize that their work was appreciated by the people with whom they worked, they developed a feeling of individual worthiness. Accordingly, a group of rather straggly, generally unacceptable workers were easily and quickly converted to valued employees.

Some department chiefs have never thought of using women in what many consider a rather strenuous job. However, the females often work out even better than the males. Most stretchers and wheelchairs are not difficult to move and the movement of patients from a bed to a stretcher or from a chair to a wheelchair is not done alone by the messenger. The females present a less threatening appearance to the patient, and the female personality is frequently more pleasant. There can be no doubt that the patients relate to the women better than to young boys. Furthermore, an older woman working in such a capacity is usually well motivated or she would not be there. Turnover from the job is close to zero, and the messenger job often serves as a stepping stone to higher positions within a department.

The first step in obtaining messengers for the radiology department is to determine how many are needed. The number of inpatients per day is ascertained and an estimate is then made of the number of patients required on the floor per hour. One has to make the somewhat inaccurate assumption that the number of patients is constant throughout the day, i.e. that the same number of patients should be brought to the floor every hour of the day. Most patients seen in the morning are those requiring lengthy examinations, such as intravenous urography and gastrointestinal fluoroscopy, while the patients in the afternoon frequently require lesser amounts of time on the floor. It must be realized that the inpatient workload is directly influenced by the number of messengers and radiographic examinations cannot be performed if the patients cannot be brought to the floor. The number of messengers and number of patients required per hour on the floor will also serve as a guide to work flow for outpatients. It is those times during the day when it is not possible to have adequate numbers of inpatients in the radiology department, perhaps at lunchtime, when outpatient work should be performed.

The important determinant is the length of time it takes a messenger to leave the radiology floor and return with a patient. In most hospitals it takes an average of ten minutes for a messenger to leave the radiology department, take an elevator to the patient's room, see that the patient is in a stretcher or wheelchair, take the elevator back down to the radiology department, and deliver the patient. This takes into account time spent waiting for delayed elevators or for the floor to have the patient ready. If indeed it takes ten minutes to bring the patient to the floor, it will also take ten minutes to return the same patient. In other words, each patient will require approximately twenty minutes of a messenger's time, with each messenger only retrieving three patients per hour. Accordingly, if the messenger works eight hours per day, each messenger can bring only approximately twenty-five patients to the floor. If a department requires one hundred inpatients, that department will require four messengers.

Another consideration is the method of transportation which will be used to bring patients to the floor. For example, in a group of approximately 300 consecutive inpatients requiring chest examinations, 43 percent walked to the department while wheelchairs were used for 36 percent of the patients and stretchers for 21 percent. It goes without saying that the department should have adequate numbers of stretchers and wheelchairs to meet the demand.

The method by which the messenger is dispatched to the patient is also important. With a "no speak" technique, it is not necessary for anyone to tell the messenger anything. This does away with one area of potential difficulty, misunderstanding or misinterpretation of verbal instructions. The "no speak" technique hinges on index cards on which the patient's name and location are typed by the receptionist. The control officer calls the patient's floor approximately fifteen minutes before the patient is needed, explains that the department is ready for the patient, and finds out how he or she will travel. The control officer then writes the method of transportation on the index card and places it in either the in-coming or out-going box so that the messenger readily can see it. It should be added that waiting space for the messengers must be made available near the control officer. The messenger takes the card from the incoming box, fills in the messenger log (as illustrated in Fig. 6), and puts down his or her initials, the patient's name, the floor, and the time of departure. When the messenger returns he or she again fills in the time. At the time that the messengers select the cards from the incoming box, they also look at the outgoing box. If there are cards for patients to be returned from the radiology department to the floors they will also take those cards. In this fashion they are not empty handed either in going or in coming from the department.

Figure 6

MESSENGER LOG BOOK

Messenger	Patient	Location	Time	Time
Name	Name		Left	Returned

The logbook plays many roles. It is readily available to the control officer who can quickly determine if a patient has been brought to the floor or if a patient has been taken back from the floor. The log book also serves to keep track of the messengers. Obviously, a messenger who went to bring a patient to the department at 1:00 p.m. should be back before 3:00 p.m. Other useful information is available from the logbook. For example, if it is seen that whenever a messenger goes to the fifth floor to retrieve a patient that the time involved is twice as long as when the messenger goes to any other floor within the hospital, there is a problem on the fifth floor. The logbook provides hard data with which to discuss this problem with the fifth floor nursing personnel.

The messenger situation can be summarized as follows:
1. The radiology department must have its own messenger service.
2. Females are as suitable, if not more so, than males in this job category.
3. One messenger can handle three patients per hour.
4. A card system in conjunction with a logbook sign-out and sign-in system offers a method of control.

CHAPTER 4

THE RADIOLOGICAL EXAMINATION

NEXT to the radiologist, the radiological technologist is the *most important* person in the radiology department. This is the individual who performs the examinations and upon whom the radiologist relies to present him with quality films upon which he can make medical determinations.

The technologists are also the most abused persons in the radiology department. In addition to performing the functions for which they are trained, they are also called upon to be janitors, patient movers, and dispatchers, and to perform many other jobs. This is the classical example of the failure of the administrator to see that each job is funneled down to a person who has appropriate training for the job, the Partition-Responsibility Theory. There can be no doubt that there is great waste of the technologist's time in most departments and that the technologist is providing an expensive form of labor to perform many tasks that could be well done by other less trained individuals.

The appropriate number of technologists for a department is frequently a point of dispute with the hospital administration, and this subject can be approached from many points of view. Most hospitals seem to require at least 1½ technologists per radiographic room. While it is true that some rooms can be adequately run with a single technologist, there are times during the day, such as morning fluoroscopy, where two technologists per room are mandatory. Furthermore, during lunch hours, coffee breaks, etc. additional personnel must be available. It should be noted that no consideration is given to the use of student technologists. The students are present for educational purposes and, although permitted to fully participate in activities of the department, they should not be counted upon to carry out the routine workload of the department.

In addition to a minimum of 1½ technologists per room, other technological personnel are required. Among these are a chief, an assistant chief, a student supervisor, and technologists for nighttime and weekend coverage. These figures assume that the department is open twenty-four hours a day 365 days of a year, and that the evening workload requires three technologists while the midnight shift requires only one. The requirements on the weekend will be determined by the workload; in most departments the twenty-four hour workload on Saturday and Sunday is approximately one half of a routine workday. Accordingly, several additional technologists will be required. The numbers of technologists of the department at St. Vincent Hospital are shown in Table I.

TABLE I

STAFF TECHNOLOGISTS

Weekdays			Weekends - Saturday and Sunday	
8 A.M. - 5 P.M.	16		4 T X 8 hr X 2 D =	64 hr
5 P.M. - 12 A.M.	4		3 T X 8 hr X 2 D =	48 hr
12 A.M. - 8 A.M.	1		1 T X 8 hr X 2 D =	16 hr
				128 hr or
				3 technologists

Total staff technologists twenty-four + administrator, chief and assistant, and educational coordinator.

It is frequently a difficult problem to assign technologists to evening and weekend coverage. It is preferable to have separate individuals working these shifts rather than rotating the routine daytime people. Most technologists prefer not to work nights and weekends, and it is a great incentive to work in a department in which they are not called upon to do so. On the other hand, many technologists *do* prefer to work these shifts, and there are certain incentives. The first of these is money, and night and weekend people should earn significantly more (at least 25%) for working during these time periods. Some technologists prefer to work these shifts because their work periods are so well stabilized since they never have to rotate to other shifts.

The author has tried several other techniques. For example, one technologist who works on a sixteen hour shift (8 A.M. — 11

P.M.) on Saturday and Sunday, and who qualified as a full-time employee by spending an additional eight-hour period in the department sometime during the week. Flexible work schedules have also been tried, such as a Wednesday through Sunday night or a Friday through Tuesday night shift.

Few people realize how little of the technologist's time is spent performing radiological examinations. This does not mean that the technologist is not working as hard as possible during the work period. It means, rather, that the department is not run in an efficient manner which would make it possible for the technologist to perform more radiographic examinations. In most departments, the technologist spends approximately 30 percent of his or her time taking films! If it were possible to double this figure so that the technologist spent 60 percent of his or her time taking films, the department's workload could be doubled without the addition of a single machine or room to the department. The technologists' problem is either that patients are not made readily available to them, or that they must spend large amounts of time performing tasks other than the taking of x rays. Among these are the washing of appliances, developing films, the transportation of patients, etc.

This point can be easily checked if a sheet is placed in each radiographic room and the technologist is asked to fill in the type of examination and the times that the patient entered and left the room for each examination during a given day. Analysis of these figures will quickly demonstrate the amount of time in which the room is occupied with patients. Once these figures are available, it is a simple matter to discuss with the technologist why so little time was spent obtaining films. The technologists are usually able to identify quickly the commitments on their time other than the performance of x-ray examinations and the obstructions within the department which are an encumbrance.

Another subject worthy of consideration is subspecialization of x-ray technologists. In many departments the technologist is perpetually rotated between rooms on a daily, weekly, or monthly basis. The author prefers to permanently assign technologists to certain rooms. There is no doubt that the technologist can perform the examination better and more efficiently if he or she is doing the same type of examination all the time. Furthermore the technologist becomes quite familiar with the room and the procedure. The technologists themselves develop a certain sense of pride in their work. While it is true that all technologists can perform intravenous urograms, it is also true that some technologists can do the examination more quickly and better than others. Not all technologists prefer to be subspecialized and it is not mandatory that they do so. Within each department there are enough technologists who would like to subspecialize that at least one permanent technologist can be assigned to each subspecialty area while the others rotate on a monthly basis. Another advantage of a permanent assignment is that it makes it possible to delegate authority within the department. One disadvantage of the system is that, as the technologists superspecialize, they become less familiar in obtaining examinations of other types. For this reason, the presence of rotators is beneficial.

In addition to assigning the technologist, attention must be given to the equipment within the room. All radiographic rooms must be cross calibrated with one another and although this goal is readily attainable, it has not been met in most departments. Cross calibration is mandatory if films of equal density are to be obtained throughout the department. While the equipment may be of various manufacturers or vintage, it is possible to insure that equivalent radiographs are obtained from each machine in the department at given settings. The equipment in a department may be quite old and antiquated, but it is possible to accomplish this goal through the careful supervision of a physicist, and a great deal of pressure brought on the companies. It goes without saying that all machines must work properly. There is no excuse for loose knobs, broken handles, etc.

The next step is the development of technique guides; there are two types of technique charts available within the department. The first of these lists each examination and the projections and numbers of films in each examination. The chief must act as the final arbitrator between the radiologists and make the final decision as to what constitutes a uniform basic examination. (Of course each radiologist may request additional films.) This is again an example of a written protocol. There can be no doubt as to the exact numbers of films and projections in each examination which each technologist must take.

In addition, there is also a technical factor technique chart. Since all of the rooms are cross calibrated, two technique charts, one for the single phase and another for the three phase units, suffice for the entire department. Again the chief has to act as the final arbitrator to define an optimum density for a group of radiologists. All patients should be measured with calipers prior to obtaining a film. If a film of inappropriate quality is shown to the radiologist, his response is usually to ask which technique was used and whether or not the technique was from the chart. The answer to the latter question is frequently "no." The technique charts take into account the fact that most rooms are phototimed.

Throughout the department, a single type of film and a single type of screen is used; the only exception is that cardboard holders are used for extremity work. The single screen is again an attempt to simplify things as much as possible so that the technologist cannot become confused between different screens used for different examinations. While it could be argued that detail screens or screens of varying speeds have a role to play within the department, errors made in the switching from one screen to another more than compensate for any advantage of the use of these types of screens.

Finally, supplies belong in, or close to, each room. Again a written list is posted; this list is checked each morning by the technologist in charge to be sure that there are no omissions. Under this scheme, there should be no delays during the working day because of lack of supplies.

No area of the radiology department receives as little attention as the darkroom, yet here is an area of gross inefficiency. It is assumed that cassettes with films in them are used in the department, that the films must be manually fed into the processor, that unexposed film must then be placed within the cassette, and that there is one central darkroom. Dispersed darkrooms are preferable, but they do not exist in most departments. It is not at all uncommon to see long lines of technologists queued up at the darkroom waiting for their films to come out of the processor. A delay in film processing may act as a major impediment to rapid patient flow within the department.

One of the first decisions that has to be made concerns the person who will work in the darkroom. Who will feed the films into the processor and change the cassettes? In all too many departments the technologist who has taken the film is the one who will perform this function. This is a waste of the technologist's time, and it is an inappropriate use of his or her talent and ability. While the technologists are at the processor they cannot simultaneously be performing examinations in their radiographic rooms. Darkroom aides can be utilized for this function, and the increased productivity on the part of the radiographic technologist more than compensates for the additional salaries required for the darkroom aide. This again demonstrates the principle of delegation of work and assigning each function to the proper job level.

It is often possible to use the physically handicapped, especially the blind, in the darkroom. This is a job which they are often able to perform better than people with sight. (A sighted person should, however, be included in the darkroom crew.) Another important consideration is an assignment of a priority schedule to the processors. It will usually work out that certain examinations can best be lumped together by being fed through the same processor rather than by being handled on a hit or miss basis. Part of the decision rests on the frequency of the type of examinations, the number of films, and the time of day that the examination is performed. For example, the priority rating for a department that performs gastrointestinal fluoroscopy only in the mornings must take into account that there will be no gastrointestinal fluoroscopic films in the afternoon. Equally obvious, a gastrointestinal series with perhaps seven or eight films must be weighed against the chest film which requires only two films. Account must also be taken for long runs of special procedure films. For example, a processor is usually tied up for at least twenty minutes when a full angiographic series is fed through it, and it would be inappropriate for other examinations to be held back waiting for that processor to be free. Although an angiographic series is not fed through the processor frequently each day, special plans will have to be made for the times when it is.

Figures show that a darkroom aide can handle only about thirty films per hour. At St. Vincent Hospital, which at one time had only three processors, about eight gastrointestinal series were performed each hour and this presented a real problem. Assuming an average of seven films per gastrointestinal series, approximately fifty-six films per hour had to be processed for the gastrointestinal suite alone. Using the calculation of thirty films per hour, two processors had to be set aside for gastrointestinal fluoroscopy. This left the third processor to handle the remainder of the department. It worked out that the darkroom aide could actually feed about forty-five films. Accordingly, the overflow from the single remaining processor could be handled at times in one of the two processors otherwise devoted to gastrointestinal fluoroscopy. After 11 A.M. when fluoroscopy was usually completed, the processor situation was no longer a problem.

Another consideration is the person who will check the films for quality at the end of the processor, and a variety of possibilities exist. In many departments, a radiologist is assigned to the end of the processor, and either checks the films or gives a final dictation as they come out of the processor. It is difficult to convince many radiologists that they should function under these adverse working conditions, although this method does work quite well in some departments. If the radiologists is not to do the job, it must be done by a technologist, and one choice would be the technologist who performed the examination. However, this means that he or she would be waiting at the end of the machine until the films came out, and that authority for film quality would be delegated among many individuals. The use of a quality control technologist (QQT) eliminates these problems. This individual should be someone who has a greater than usual knowledge of film technique. The QQT checks all films that come out of the processor and informs a technologist if a repeat is required. At St. Vincent Hospital, the retake rate is approximately 5 percent. Some figures from a recent study are shown in Table II. The QQT also plays an important educational role in the department, advising individual technologists how to obtain better films.

The QQT is a key individual in the department. The radiologist communicates problems with film quality to the QQT who then deals with the individual technologists. (Obviously, the radiologist is also able to communicate with the individual technologists if necessary.) This system insures that all radiologists' complaints about film quality are filtered back to one individual

TABLE II

REPEATED EXAMINATIONS

Total Films - 7 Wk	23,638
Number Retakes	1,247
or 5.3%	

Reason -
Overexposed	25%
Poor Positioning	23%
Underexposed	20%
	68%

Type of Examination repeated:
Thoracic Spine	21%
Abdomen	15%
Chest	3%

rather than being diffused throughout the department. The QQT knows that he or she will hear from the radiologist if the film is of poor technical quality; at the same time, the QQT takes great pride in the film quality of the department and has an interesting and fascinating job.

Another function of the darkroom should be to place patient identification on the films, assuming that the patient's name or identifying number is not automatically placed on the film at the time of the radiographic exposure by a mechanism inherent in the equipment. Such devices are frequent in certain types of modern equipment but do not exist in most departments. A favorite technique of patient identification is the use of small lead numbers to positively mark the film at the time that the exposure is made. This system requires a surprising amount of time to select and place the numbers on the film in some sort of holder, it is expensive, and it often results in a sloppy appearance. The flash card system in which typed flashcards are placed in the darkroom with the films, is preferable. In spite of the use of blind people, it has not proved a problem in terms of identification, and film identification problems are extremely unusual. Inexpensive flashers are now available which include time clocks so that, in addition to the patient information, the time at which the film was processed is also indicated.

Calibration of the processors is also important. This is often a weak link in film quality, and regardless of the amount of care taken in obtaining the radiographic exposure, the processor will be a determining factor in film quality. Different films and processors will function best with varying combinations of chemicals. Both the film salesman and the processor solution people are knowledgeable in this area and should be encouraged to determine the best chemical combination for a given processor-film combination.

All processors must be calibrated so that they not only function identically from day to day but also function identically with each other. In a simple method of processor calibration, films are exposed using a sensitometer. Each morning a freshly exposed test film is fed through each processor by the QQT. The densities under the step wedge are then determined using a simple densitometer. Densitometers are now available which sell for approximately 200 dollars, and the investment is minuscule when compared to the value within the department. The densities under the step wedges are placed on a graph and are compared on a daily basis. If a variation is encountered, the reason must be immediately determined prior to use of the processor for the day. With this system the processors guarantee that densities are within 10 percent of the expected.

This chapter has pointed out that:
1. The radiological technologist is the most important person in the department.
2. The appropriate number of technologists for a department must be determined.
3. The technologist must be permitted to perform radiological examinations. Few if any technologists spend as much as 50 percent of their time doing this.
4. Technique charts including numbers and types of projections as well as technical factors must be used. The chief

frequently will have to act as a referee in reaching some compromise between the radiologists.

5. The darkroom should operate efficiently.
6. A single technologist, the QQT, should be assigned responsibility for insuring optimum film quality.
7. The x-ray machines and processors must be properly calibrated.

CHAPTER 5

THE FILE ROOM

$\mathbf{O}$F all the functioning units in the radiology department, there can be no doubt that the file room is the most complex, the most frustrating, the most difficult, the most perplexing, and the least efficient. The subject is so vast that it is a difficult one to discuss, but the following outline will be followed:

1. File room space
2. File room numbering systems
3. File room envelopes
4. Characterization of file room functions and distribution of personnel

SPACE

No file room has *enough* space, but a reasonable amount of space must be decided upon. The important consideration is the number of linear feet of file space available. A file rack which is five shelves tall, with each shelf approximately seventeen inches deep is rather standard; a rack with six shelves is too tall. It can be assumed that approximately forty envelopes can be filed in one foot of space. As an example, in six feet of space, assuming a five shelf file rack, 1200 jackets can be filed.

A related problem is the determination of the number of jackets which should be kept in the main radiology department. Obviously, the more the better, but a minimum of one year's films is adequate. In a room sixteen by thirty-five feet, it is possible to place 450 linear ft. of shelves and still permit adequate working space for personnel. This space is adequate to hold approximately seven months of films, or approximately 18,000 jackets. During a one-month period at St. Vincent Hospital, calls were received for 4350 jackets; 2200 of these were in the active file, while 1200 represented new numbers. In other words 78 percent of the departments needs were satisfied by the active file. Another 3½ yr of films are stored in a basement file room; these provide an additional 700 jackets. Only 3 percent of the department's inquiries were for films which were older than four years. Figures from another survey conducted in our department are shown in Table III.

TABLE III

AVAILABILITY OF OLD FILMS

117 Day Period		
Number of Patients	3114	
Number of Readmissions	2508	
within 1 year	2071	83%
within 3 year	2312	.92%
within 5 year	2424	97%
within 7 year	2473	99%
within 9 year	2495	99%

Another pressing question concerns the length of time that x-ray films should be maintained. In most states there are no laws dictating this figure, but many malpractice lawyers suggest five or six years as a reasonable length of time. Unfortunately, there are a number of cases in which the old films would contribute significantly to a patient's medical care. In the case of a patient with a solitary lung nodule whose five-year-old films have been destroyed, the absence of old films may well mean that the patient will have to undergo a thoracotomy. It must be realized that the hospital space is quite costly, and that it is probably inappropriate for the radiologist to feel that a large amount of space can be provided to his department within the main hospital building. However, most hospitals have additional buildings with partially vacated basements. Those that do not have such facilities frequently are located in cities that have old abandoned warehouses, garages, or supermarkets. Rental of such space is frequently less than one dollar per square foot. It should be realized that the space need not be heated and that lighting can be very minimal. Furthermore, wood shelving (assuming that fire laws will permit it) can be constructed by hospital personnel at a minimal cost. This depository can be visited once or twice a day or every other day and can fill the needs of the department for a large film depository.

A word should be said about microfilming and its use. At the time that this book is being written, the small films still leave something to be desired in technical quality, and though impressive figures can be produced showing that file room space may be diminished by more than 90 percent using microfilm, it should be recalled that the current price is $.15 per exposure. The cost of the equipment is at least $50,000. In a department doing 50,000 examinations per year, assuming three films are taken for each examination and that films are kept for five years, amortization of the equipment adds another $6.70 per film so that the total cost per exposure is $21.70. The above costs do not allow for space and personnel required to make the copies. The reduction in cost assuming immediate destruction of the large films with significant amounts of silver reclaimed, has also been omitted.

In order to calculate the cost of maintaining 750,000 large films for five years, we would assume storing forty-eight films per foot in an area of 1432 square ft, with five-foot high shelving, 2½ ft aisles, and 1½ ft shelf depth. If the cost of using the space is figured at five dollars per square foot, and the cost of shelving at twenty fivs cents per running inch, the total cost of storing each film works out to $5.80 per film, approximately 25 percent the cost of microfilm. The formula used to derive the above numbers are shown in Figure 7.

Figure 7

DERIVATION OF COST FOR STANDARD SHELVING

Cost of Space:

$$\frac{4 \text{ folders/in X 2 exams/folder X 3 films/exam X 12 in X 5 shelves high}}{1 \text{ ft X 1.5 ft depth/shelf X } \frac{1}{2} \text{ aisle X 2.5 ft/aisle}} = 523.6 \text{ Films/ft}^2$$

$$\frac{\$5/\text{ft}^2/\text{yr X 5 yr}}{523.6 \text{ films /ft}^2} = 4.8 \text{¢/film}$$

Cost of shelving:

$$\frac{150,000 \text{ films/yr X 5 yr}}{4 \text{ folders/in X 2 exam/folder X 3 films/exam}} \text{ X \$0.25/in shelving} = \$7813$$

$$\frac{\$7813}{150,000 \text{ films X 5 yr}} = 1 \text{ ¢/film}$$

$$4.8¢ + 1.0¢ = 5.8¢$$

Size of File Room:

$$\frac{150,000 \text{ films/yr X 5 yr}}{523.6 \text{ films/ft}^2} = 1432 \text{ ft}^2$$

Another alternative might be the use of mobile shelving. Assuming costs of such shelving to be between fifty cents and one dollar per inch, and assuming a 30 percent reduction is required in space, the five-year cost per film is slightly more than when regular shelving is used. (Fig. 8) Of course, in this system, one also has to worry about personnel getting crushed between shelves. Comparative annual costs are summarized in Table IV. The reader should realize that these cost comparisons are only approximations. If one were to apply this sort of reasoning to one's own situation, one would insert more accurate figures corresponding to their local situation. In addition, one would take into account the cost of personnel involved, the timing of silver reclamation, the cost of space saved, etc. Furthermore, it should be appreciated that there may be some situations in which adequate space for the use of regular shelving for storage just is not available, and that one may be forced to use another system.

Figure 8

DERIVATION OF COST FOR MOVEABLE SHELVING

Cost of Space:

4.8¢/film (cost for standard shelving) X 70% (moveable savings) = 3.4¢ film

Cost of Shelving:

$$\frac{150{,}000 \text{ films X } 5 \text{ yr}}{4 \text{ folders/in X } 2 \text{ exams/ folder X } 3 \text{ films/exam}} \text{ X } 0.77¢/\text{in shelving} = \$24{,}063$$

$$\frac{\$24{,}063}{150{,}000 \text{ films X } 5 \text{ yr}} = 3.2¢/\text{film}$$

3.4¢ + 3.2¢ = 6.6¢/film

TABLE IV

COMPARISON OF ANNUAL FILM STORAGE COSTS

	Per Film	Total
Conventional	5.8¢	$8700
Moveable	6.6¢	$9900
Microfilm	21.7¢	$32,550

NUMBERING SYSTEMS

Unfortunately, many departments still adhere to the consecutive numbering system, a system that begins with the number 1 and consecutively numbers things to 100,000, 1,000,000 etc. Using this system, no color coding is used, and it is impossible to identify a jacket without carefully examining the number written or printed on the jacket. Let us assume that at the beginning of the year the first number used was 1 and at the end of the year the number 10,000 was reached. The following year, one began at 10,001 and reached the number 17,000. During each succeeding year fewer numbers are activated during that time period. Eventually, some sort of purging of the main file room will have to be done so that the previous year's jackets can be moved to another file room to make additional space available for the new patients. Each jacket will have to be scrutinized to find the date of the last exam. Some of the older consecutive numbers will be removed while those of patients who have had films within the last year will be left behind. There are then gaps on the shelves and all films must be backshifted to make room for the new envelopes.

Under this system, the area of the file room with the latest numbers requires more frequent use than the area of earliest numbers. Furthermore, as stated above, about 20 percent of the older numbered jackets that have been purged, because they had not been used for a year, will be reactivated. These older jackets will now have to be squeezed into the shelves in the proper consecutive order, and no matter how much space has been left for this contingency, it is never enough. The main disadvantages of this system, therefore, are that it is impossible to identify or age film jackets without looking directly at them, that the film jackets change places on the shelves from time to time, that considerable shifting of large numbers of jackets is frequently required, and that the whole system frequently breaks down.

The terminal digit system makes use of the fact that all numbers, regardless of their length, must end in one of 100 combinations, i.e. 00 — 99. For example, numbers 1 to 100,000 can be equally divided into 100 parts, with 1000 numbers in each terminal digit subdivision. Given a series of patients, the law of averages states that an almost equal number will fall into each terminal digit. If the available linear footage of filing space is divided by 100, an equal amount of space is assigned to each terminal digit. A given terminal digit will always remain in the same place in the file room, so that the file room personnel know exactly where to go when looking for a number with a specific terminal digit. Under the consecutive numbering system, as stated above, a film ending in a given number can be anywhere throughout the file room.

The system can be further modified by selecting out the fourth digit from the end, i.e. the thousand digit, and this will be referred to as the middle digit. For example, given the number 123456, 56 are the terminal digits and 3 is the middle digit. In other words, within each terminal digit, films can be subdivided into ten further compartments by using the thousand digit as a middle digit marker. As shown in the example, all films with the same middle and terminal digit are found in the same section of the file room.

Another benefit of the system is the ease with which numbers can now be remembered. Given the number 123456 the file room personnel under a consecutive numbering system must remember the number in exactly that order. However, under a terminal digit system, the automatic tendency is to divide the numbers into units of two so that the number would be remembered as 56 34 12. The file room personnel begin looking for the case by going immediately to the 56 section and that particular number will be one of the relatively few jackets found there. If 100,000 numbers are used, the largest possible amount of jackets that could be present with the terminal digit of 56 would be 1000. Using the middle digit 3, now reduces the number of possibilities to ten. In reality, there will usually be no more than fifteen to twenty jackets per middle terminal digit combination. In an active file of 17,000 jackets, there are an average of eighteen jackets per middle-terminal digit. The greatly reduced time required by file room personnel to find a film should be obvious.

The middle and terminal digit systems are now modified by the addition of color coding. It must be appreciated that ten colors will make it possible to identify all numbers within a system. The present color coding scheme in use at St. Vincent Hospital is shown in Table V. For example, a number ending in 00 would be red — red. Broad bands of tape are provided, or envelopes can be preprinted with the terminal digit already printed on the ends of the jackets; the appropriate colored tape for the middle digit is added when the jacket is first used. The three colors, i.e. the middle and two terminal digit numbers, can be identified from across the room and reduce the possible choices by the file room personnel to approximately fifteen envelopes. Furthermore, it is virtually impossible to misfile under this system. For example all of the 00 or red — red jackets are in a line on the filing shelf. If one sees a red — red jacket elsewhere in the file room, it will disturb the row of colors in which it sits. The corollary is the fact that no other colors can appear in the red — red row.

TABLE V

COLOR CODE

0	Red	5	Black
1	Grey	6	Yellow
2	Blue	7	Brown
3	Orange	8	Pink
4	Purple	9	Green

Examples: 123456 - orange, black, yellow

159500 - green, red, red

There is a certain reluctance and hesitancy on the part of radiologists and file room personnel to convert from the consecutive number system to the terminal digit system with the feeling that the terminal digit system may be too complex for the personnel to comprehend. However, a file room clerk with average intelligence can be taught the new system within thirty minutes, and personnel that have worked under both systems readily admit that the terminal digit system is far superior. Another hesitancy is the effort required in the physical act of conversion. It should be noted that the companies which sell the terminal digit envelopes provide consultation on this subject, will plan the redistribution of the file room space, and will help plan the actual conversion move.

ENVELOPES

The design of the film envelopes is important. The envelope should be of sturdy stock, at least eleven point weight. It should be of proper size so that it fits on the file room shelving and easily accepts x-ray films. The envelope can open from the side or top although the top loading envelope is preferable, as is an envelope with expanding sides so that it can easily handle those patients that require multiple x-ray examinations.

The major envelope in which all films belonging to a given patient are placed is referred to as the master folder. On the front of the envelope, in addition to the patient's name and unit number there should also be some wide lines on which are placed the date, the number of films, and the name of examination performed. There also should be in bold letters the statement *Master Folder Must Never Leave the X-Ray Department;* if films leave the department they should be placed in special envelopes called loan folders. It should be noted that it is possible to place printing on the back of the folder as well as the front; although it is better to leave the back of the envelope blank except for the x-ray number.

The end of the envelope is used for color coding. The envelopes are preprinted with the last two terminal digits in color. These arrive from the factory in boxes of 200 with four terminal digits to each box. This permits fifty envelopes of each terminal digit number to be stored on the floor at any time. As any particular terminal digit is used up, additional jackets for that number are easily requisitioned from the warehouse. Above the preprinted two-color terminal digit code is a box where a broad piece of tape is placed to denote the middle digit. This is done as the patient's name is written on the envelope. Also preprinted in color on each envelope is a thin color strip representing the last number of the current year. Below this is a blank strip where a color tape is placed indicating the month. If one has to purge the active file every seventh month, it is then a relatively simple thing to identify the month in which the examination has been performed and to move the films to the basement storage facility. Other colored coded tapes could be used to indicate patients who have died or cases which should be saved for the teaching collection or museum, etc.

Films can be further segregated within the master folder by organ system, and within each master folder it is possible for a total of six subspecialty folders to be present. These also are color coded as follows: chest — brown; G.I. — gray; bone — yellow; G.U. — orange; special procedure — green; previous films — white. For example, all chest films will be placed in the brown envelope, all G.I. exams in the gray envelope, etc. A word of explanation is necessary about the previous studies envelope. It is too great a burden to segregate the patient's previous films into the subspecialty folders when the patient's old jacket is first updated into a new folder. Therefore, all of the previous films are simply placed into the "previous" folder rather than trying to segregate them into the other subspecialty folders.

The subspecialty folder filing system has many advantages. Most radiologists have spent a good deal of time going through a thick folder containing 100 films looking for the single film of the right wrist. Under this system, all one would have to do is select the yellow envelope to locate the appropriate bone films. The system is equally appealing to the practitioner, who is also saved the effort of looking through the entire pile of films when looking for one type of examination. The system may not work all of the time, and one is dependent on the cooperation of everyone using the patient's films to see that the appropriate films find their way back into the proper envelopes. Cooperation is superb among everyone as all benefit from the system; the proper film is found in the appropriate subspecialty envelope in more than eight out of ten cases.

There are other systems of segregating films within the envelopes such as segregating each examination in a separate envelope by date, but this is awkward and bulky. It must be appreciated that the subspecialty envelopes do take up space in themselves and will cut down on the total filing space. It is estimated that they cause a reduction of approximately 10 percent but it is well worth it.

The x-ray reports should go into a special consultation folder which is then placed inside the master folder. While it is true that if one loses the master folder, one loses the x-ray report also, there is a great advantage in not having a separate filing system for the x-ray reports; the reports can always be found in the medical record.

The third type of folder as mentioned previously is the loan folder. This should be of distinctly different color than the master folder. Printed on the front of this folder should be the patient's name and number as well as a statement, again in bold letters, *These Films Should Be Returned to The X-Ray Department in 24 Hours.*

FILE ROOM FUNCTIONS AND DIVISION OF LABOR

File room operations can be divided as follows:
1. Obtaining previous jacket or the making up of a new folder.
2. Integrating a new examination into the master folder.
3. Delivering the films to the radiologist for interpretation.
4. Refiling the master folder in the main file.
5. Refiling of the x-ray reports into the master folder.
6. Finding films for clinicians and loaning them out.

Each of these functions will now be discussed in order. There should be a minimum of delay from the time the radiographic examination is obtained until it reaches the radiologist's desk for interpretation. Unfortunately in many departments it may take several hours or days to integrate the new films with the patient's previous examinations. The defect is easily explainable when it is realized that most file room personnel have no advance notice system that a patient is having a new examination and that they must have a jacket ready for these films. It is mandatory that the file room be notified of the necessity of an old jacket or preparing a new one as soon as the radiology department knows that the patient is to undergo an x-ray examination. This function should be assigned to one person, the "getter." If the x-ray requisitions on most of the inpatients and many of the outpatients are available by 8 P.M. of the previous evening, it is a simple task to have a nighttime person find the old jackets and place them in one portion of the file room. During the day, the file room can be instantly notified when the department first receives any other x-ray requisitions, and one person has the sole responsibility of finding the old jacket or making up a new jacket and placing it in this same temporary file. This function is separate and distinct from the integration of the new films into the patient's master folder.

The next step is the actual integration function. The person who performs this activity is a "setter-upper." He or she receives the new films within ten minutes after they are taken and is seated near the temporary file where the patient's old jacket or new folder has been placed. The "setter-upper" finds the appropriate jacket, records on the jacket the date and the examination which has been performed, and places the jacket with films into a separate section from whence they will be taken to the radiologist. One individual can set up approximately 200 cases per day, if the old and new jackets are readily available.

The "setter-upper" writes down the name of each patient after films have been prepared for interpretation. When the clinician wants to see films on a patient, the "setter-upper" can then readily determine if those films have been received, if they have been set up for the day, and if they have already left the film room.

Another individual must deliver the films to the radiologist. The time of delivery will be determined by the method of interpretation used in the department which is discussed in a separate chapter. It should be emphasized, however, that some ground rules must be established. These may state, for example, that the films must be delivered to the radiologist every thirty minutes, or that no more than ten cases should accumulate in the file room before they are delivered to the radiologist. This function can be carried out by an individual in addition to other functions.

Eventually, the master folders must be refiled into the main files. This function is frequently divided among several people since it is a job that is done infrequently during the day. An alternative is to have this function performsd by the nighttime person.

This same person is the one that refiles the x-ray reports into the main jacket, and this is a good example of how to estimate manpower needs. If one assumes that it takes approximately two minutes to pick up an x-ray report from a pile, to go to the main files, and to pull the master folder from the shelf, and another two minutes to place the report into the report folder and then into the master folder, one can say that it takes four minutes to refile each report folder. If one is dealing with 200 reports per day this means that it will require 800 min or 13½ work-hours of straight labor, excluding coffee, lunch hours, etc. In other words, this single function requires two people per day.

There is nothing more frustrating to the clinician than to have to line up outside the window of the file room and wait ten minutes before someone comes along to find films on his patient. Because of this, one person can be assigned to do this job, the "loaner-outer." He or she keeps a list of films that are loaned out or given to clinicians to see within the department and also receives all films that are returned to the file room by the clinicians.

While it is true that many departments refuse to sign films out, this is not really fair to the clinician. As mentioned above, a separate loan folder can be used. Once the films are signed out, the master folder is placed in an out-guide which is made of red plastic, and this is filed into the appropriate space in the master file. These out-guides are checked on a weekly basis, and if the films have not been returned, the clinicians are called. It should be noted that in most departments, there is no system of checking for films that have been signed out of the department, and the department is not usually aware of the absence of films until the films are called for. Obviously, this can create difficulty. This problem can be handled by having the clinicians fill out a slip similar to one in a library before the films are signed out. An alternate system is to keep these out-guides in a separate file that can be checked at appropriate intervals. This can be a time consuming function but a very helpful one for insuring that the maximum number of films are in the radiology department.

It is now possible to estimate the number of people required to staff the day shift of a file room dealilng with 200 new examinations per day. A minimum of a supervisor, "setter upper," "loaner outer," "old film getter," and two jacket and report filers will be needed. These six individuals must be supplimented by at least two other persons in the viewing room as described in the next chapter. At least one additional person will be required for the night shift.

The file room operation demonstrates many basic principles of management, including the specification of the distinct jobs, assignment of specific people to specific tasks, and estimation of manpower needs. Each person has a well-described job. Furthermore, if there is a delay in the films reaching the radiologist for interpretation, the exact cause of delay, whether it be the inability to obtain the old jacket or the inability to integrate the new examination with the old films, can be precisely identified.

However, in practice there is almost no delay in the films reaching the radiologist, and more importantly, there is almost no film loss. (Naturally, the only persons permitted in the file room are the file room employees.)

Rarely does anything operate at 90 percent efficiency. In a file room doing 200 examinations per day, it can be assumed that 200 folders will be pulled, films will be integrated into 200 jackets, 200 jackets will be returned to the master file, and 100 other calls will be made for films. Allowing for other usage and assuming that the jackets are used 900 times during the day and that the file room is operating at 90 percent efficiency, this means that eighty-one jackets cannot be found, a disastrous situation!

In this chapter:

1. Methods of determining needed space are given.
2. The terminal digit, color coded filing system is recommended and described.
3. Three types of film jackets, master, subspecialty, and loan, are described.
4. Specific functions within the file room and distribution of personnel are suggested.

CHAPTER 6

FILM INTERPRETATION

FILMS are interpreted in a central viewing room using multiple view boxes. Many radiologists spend only slightly more than 50 percent of their viewing time interpreting films, with the remainder of their time devoted to functions that could have been done by others, such as finding films in envelopes, placing them on view boxes, removing them, etc. The multiple view box solves this problem.

Basically, the films are placed on multiple view boxes by paramedical personnel; one person can handle 100 cases per day. A high school student can be taught within several days how to place most films up correctly (excluding fluoroscopic spot films). The same individual can remove the films from the view boxes. At the time the present examination is placed on the view box, the last similar study can also be placed with it. By this one simple maneuver it is possible to almost double the amount of the most expensive commodity in the radiology department, namely the radiologist's time.

Not only is the radiologist saved considerable amounts of time, but the clinician also benefits. At St. Vincent Hospital, there are eight multiple view boxes, each of which contains eighty, fourteen by seventeen inch viewing panels. Once the films are placed on the view boxes, they are not removed until late in the afternoon. The clinicians and house officers know that if they arrive in the department on the same day that the examination is performed that they can completely bypass the main file room and directly enter the viewing room. When they do so, they are approached by the paramedical personnel who leads them to the appropriate view box.

The eight view boxes have been subdivided as follows: Three are used for fluoroscopic examinations, one for intravenous urograms, and one for special procedures. The remaining three view boxes receive all other types of films which are placed alphabetically. If a patient has more than one type of examination, they are preferentially placed on the G.I. view box, intravenous urogram view box, and the alphabetical view boxes, in that order.

When the films are placed on the view boxes, the name of the patient, his unit number, and the type of examination is kept on a sheet in front of the view box (Fig. 9). When the radiologist interprets the film, he jots down his impressions as well as his initials. The lines on the sheet correspond to the panel numbers of the view box. Under this system, it is a simple practice to double read all films, i.e. to have a second radiologist verify the impression of the original interpretor. The double reading is frequently performed quicker than the primary interpretation; however, if only one error is found during a week, it is well worth the effort.

Figure 9

VIEW BOX SHEET

Panel Number	Name	Unit Number	Interpretation	Radiologist
1.				
2.				
3.				
4.				
5.				
6.				

The master folders are kept at the view boxes and are readily available if further films are required. After the x-ray reports are signed by the radiologists, it is also a simple task to file the report folder back into the master folder before the films are returned to the main file room. This results in a great savings of time.

A radiologist is assigned to the main interpretation room at all times. He rotates from view box to view box and interprets each film as it is placed on the view box. As stated in the previous chapter, the films are not allowed to sit in the file room but are brought over to the viewing room several at a time as soon as they are set up. They are then placed on the view box so that almost immediate interpretation is possible. Likewise, the reports are typed almost immediately so that these functions take no more than an hour.

The multiple view box system also is a great aid in accelerating the interpretation of films from the night before. All films that are obtained after 5 P.M. are placed on the alternators by the nighttime personel. When the radiologists enter the department in the morning, they find the films waiting for them, properly arranged, ready for dictation. Each radiologist sits down in front of a multiple view box and the interpretation of the previous night's work, perhaps fifty or so cases, is easily completed by 8:30 A.M. by three people readily interpreting a reasonable number of films. The previous night's work is then returned to the file room.

The sheets which have been filled out by the paramedical personnel and the radiologist are given to the receptionist at the end of the day. When people call for the x-ray reports on the following day, the receptionist has a ready reference to find the report without having to find the films. If calls come in on the same day that the films are interpreted, the receptionist simply goes to the appropriate view box and finds, in writing, a simple report, so that he does not have to find the radiologist or look for the typewritten report in order to respond to the telephone caller.

A word or two should be said about the multiple view boxes available. The best panels are those that are made of glass, twenty inches tall, with rollers for holding films on both the top and bottom of each panel. In this fashion two ten-inch spot films can be placed one above the other and they are held securely in place. The glass does not warp as plastic may do secondary to heat. A view box with a broad foot pedal allows the panels to be easily changed. The number of panels per view box is worthy of consideration. While view boxes are manufactured that hold up to 200 or 300, fourteen by seventeen inch films, it should be appreciated that this will increase the number of times that the radiologist is interrupted by visiting clinicians while trying to read films. The interruptions are a consideration, but with only eighty spaces per view box, the interruptions are not a major problem.

Another consideration is the height of the view boxes, and some of them do require special ceiling heights. The author has little use for viewers with detachable carriages so that large numbers of films can be mounted elsewhere. This system is not preferred, because the author chooses to read films one at a time rather than having to wait for a large number of cases to be loaded. A final consideration is the amount of light emitted by the view box. In general, there should be individual switches for each panel.

A word or two should also be said about the dictating devise. In most departments, the radiologist holds a microphone in one of his hands and activates it with a thumb switch, but the radiologist is really better off if he has two hands free rather than one hand occupied with a microphone. It is a simple matter to arrange for a foot pedal with a neck microphone. Another consideration is whether the dictating machine will use a belt, disc, or tape. No matter how efficient one is, the three former devices do tend to get lost or confused. With a remote control system in which a ninety-minute belt or tape is in the secretaries office, the belt is never changed or seen and will hold up to ninety minutes of dictation. This system also permits the secretary to be typing one word behind the radiologist so that she can be typing the report as it is dictated. This type of system is vastly preferable to the others, is of no greater cost, and yet, for some reason, is not commonly in use.

Under this interpretation system, all master folders can be found in one of two places, either the file room or the main viewing room. If films are interpreted in offices of individual radiologists, the films may be in as many as six different places. Under the multiple view box system, all of the films are in one central location. A further advantage of the system is that all of the radiologists are in one room so they are readily available to one another and to the clinicians for consulting purposes. A disadvantage of the system is that the room can become congested and noisy.

In summary, the use of multiple view boxes saves the radiologist between one third and one half of his time. Leaving the films on display also benefits the clinician. Other advantages include the feasibility of double readings and the ease of refiling of typed reports. A central interpretation area eases film finding problems. Some suggestions about dictation equipment are also given.

CHAPTER 7

REPORT TRANSCRIPTION

AMAJOR problem in almost every radiology department is the accurate, efficient transcription of the radiographic reports. The department's goal should be to have the radiologic reports on most examinations performed each day on the patient's chart by evening.

It might be useful to consider some of the systems that are less commonly in use. The first such system is the computer processing of radiological reports. In some combination or other, the report is generated by and stored in the computer; a hard copy is provided as well. In addition to yielding a report, considerable additional information can be generated, such as cases for the teaching collection, billing information, etc. At the time that this book is being written, computer reporting is in its infancy. The cost of such a system is prohibitive, in most hospitals printers are not available at all nursing stations, and it is doubtful that very many hospitals will be using this system even ten years from now.

Another system involves the radiologist dictating directly to a secretary who is seated at a typewriter at his side and who types the report as the radiologist dictates. This system sometimes works very well, and there probably is no other manual system that will insure that the report is typed as promptly. However, the secretary's presence may slow down the dictation somewhat. Furthermore, there are times when the radiologist is not dictating and the secretary has little to do, and there are times when the radiologist wants to dictate a case and the secretary happens to be away from her desk.

The remainder of this chapter will be devoted to the system in use in most hospitals, one in which the radiologist dictates his report on some sort of recording machine and the secretary transcribes the report onto an x-ray requisition. The first question that must be answered is the number of secretaries or transcrip-

52

tionists required. A distinction should be made between a secretary and a typist. A typist is someone who is expert at transcription only and who cannot perform efficiently other secretarial tasks, such as interviewing, telephoning, scheduling, etc. Typists are frequently less costly than secretaries, and this again demonstrates the principle of filling job functions with people who are trained to do them; there is no reason to have a trained secretary who takes shorthand simply sitting behind the typewriter all day and typing.

The rate at which secretaries type is highly variable: One factor is the skill of the secretary; another is the length and complexity of the x-ray report. It is a simple matter to have each secretary keep track of the number of reports typed per day. One can then quickly make some calculations. At one time in my own department there were five secretaries doing approximately 200 reports per hour. Yet, our secretarial pool is much more efficient than many others. The results of this study and the cost per report is shown in Table VI.

TABLE VI

REPORTS

```
1000 Reports/Wk - 5 Typists - 200/Wk
40   Reports/Day or 5 Reports/Hr
$3.00/Hr X 40 Hr X 5 Typists = $600.00
Labor 1000 Reports/$600            0.600
Forms $44/1000                     0.044
Typewriter
   (leased) $70/Yr or $1.50/Wk     0.006
                                $  0.65 Each
```

The starting point in determining secretarial needs is to calculate the number of reports per hour which can be performed by each individual concerned. It is also imperative that the job assignments within the secretarial pool be perfectly clear. The pool frequently has functions other than transcription of x-ray reports. However, the transcription function is the top priority item, and other functions will just have to wait until that job is done.

Another important point that must be realized is the number of x-ray reports on a given day is finite and that it does not matter if the reports are typed on that day or five days later, the number is the same. For example, assume that there are approximately 225 x-ray reports per day which must be typed. Whether these reports are typed on Monday or Friday, the volume of work is identical. Once the secretaries realize this, and once they have caught up, there is no reason why they should not stay caught up.

Further comment is required on function priority. As stated above, the typing of x-ray reports is the first priority item. In a large secretarial pool, it may be that one person can be spared for other functions. The principle of division of job responsibilities into specific areas and the assignment of definite responsibility is again demonstrated here. One way that this can be accomplished is to assign certain secretaries to specific radiologists. If some of the secretaries have nothing to do when their radiologists are not dictating, they can help out the others. It does not matter whether these secretaries are working full time or not, as long as they are typing all of the reports of their radiologists.

A second system which can be employed in a subspecialized department is to divide the secretaries among the subspecialties. For example, one secretary was assigned to gastrointestinal, one to urinary, one to pulmonary, and one to bone sections. It was the responsibility of each to type all of the reports from that section. The total number of lines typed per day is not very different. There are other advantages to this system. The G.I. secretary becomes familiar with the radiologists doing the work in that subsection and with the terminology that is used in a particular subspecialty. An obvious advantage to the radiologist is that he is working with one secretary instead of four; he can praise the secretary when things go well, and when reports are not being typed promptly, he also knows who is responsible.

The above system can be modified with the addition of programmed magnetic typewriters. These typewriters work on the principle that a three by seven inch magnetic card is prepared as a report is typed. Typographical errors are corrected by simply back spacing and typing over them. The magnetic card will only show the latest letters, and not the mistake. It is then placed in a "reader," and a fresh report is automatically generated by the typewriter, letter perfect at a rate of 160 words per minute. It is estimated that the time saved by permitting the secretary to type at rough draft speed is greater than 30 percent.

The major use of the typewriters has been in the preparation of negative reports which amount to approximately 50 percent of our volume. While some radiologists prefer to simply indicate on the requisition that the examination is negative (a 1-word report), a longer report seems desirable. At St. Vincent Hospital there are now twenty-six programmed negative reports. At the time of dictation of the case instead of giving the usual dictation, the radiologist states the patient's name, unit number, examination and says "negative report please." He frequently will sign the blank report at that time meaning that he will never see the report again and that this will accelerate the system. Furthermore, the secretary can manually type in any additional phrases indicated by the radiologist. The secretary, instead of typing the report, simply places it in one of the special typewriters, activates the reader, and receives a perfectly typed report.

The typewriters can also be used in the preparation of positive reports. The preprogrammed function is ignored and the machine is used as a standard typewriter. As described above, the transcriptionist types the report on continuous form paper at a maximum rate of speed without erasing any typographical errors. A separate mag card is prepared as each report is typed. The cards and blank requisitions are placed in corresponding piles; the continuous form paper is discarded. At appropriate intervals, the transcriptionist stops typing, places the corresponding card in the reader and requisition in the typewriter, and produces letter perfect reports as the final product. Although it might seem that there is duplication of effort, the typographically perfect reports are generated at a much faster rate than is possible using standard electric typewriters.

The cost of the preprogrammed typewriters can often be compensated by decreasing the size of the typing pool. The facility and efficiency with which the new system works, plus the lack of typographical errors, are other justifications for its use. A recent analysis is shown in Table VII.

TABLE VII

REPORT TRANSCRIPTION

2 girls - 5 days

900 Reports - 7200 lines - 8 lines/report

1 girl - 90 Reports/day or 11.25 reports/hr

The secretaries have been instructed to type the reports as quickly as they are dictated. They must collect all undictated reports at least every hour; it is assumed that the secretary is no more than one hour behind, and this is indeed the case. Following transcription of the report, there must not be a delay in the signing of the report by the radiologist. This is another area in which the radiologist is frequently delinquent. The transcriptionists should be instructed to personally find the radiologist, and to place the requisitions in his hands. Although the radiologist at times resents this intrusion on his privacy or this distraction from other tasks, he quickly learns that this is a mandatory step if the reports are to reach the floor rapidly.

Following signing, the requisitions are separated and are placed in piles by nursing stations. It takes no more than one-half hour for a radiology department secretary to hand carry the piles of reports to each nursing station within a large hospital, rather than use the slower inhospital mail service.

A word should also be said about the forms on which the secretaries type the reports. While blank continuous form paper or special radiology department stationary can be used, it is preferable to use one of the sheets of the original x-ray request requisition filled out by the clinician.

One type of consultation request consists of a seven-part form. The top three half sheets are used for hospital billing, the control officer, and preliminary notification of the file room, respectively. The typewritten report appears on the next four sheets which belong to the patient's hospital record, the x-ray master folder, the referring physician, and the radiologist's billing office. The advantage of this system is that both the examination requested and the clinical information provided by the clinician in his own handwriting appear on the final report with the radiologist's interpretation.

In summary, the number of needed secretaries in a department must be determined. The reports should be divided between the secretaries in such a manner that definite responsibility for productivity can be assigned. The secretaries must understand that there is a finite number of reports and that the number of reports from a given day will be the same whether they are typed on that day or one week later. Finally, it is recommended that the reports be promptly signed by the radiologist and that they be hand carried to the patient floors.

CHAPTER 8

EPILOGUE

IT should be again stressed that the organizational structure of a radiology department is of utmost importance if the patient is to receive optimal care, and if the radiologist is to service to a ripe old age. Assuming that the reader has obtained at least one good idea from the previous pages and is about to undertake some reorganizational steps in his department, the following guidelines are offered which may serve him well in his hour of need. The following paragraphs are not original, but have been passed down throughout the ages.

You're an Optimist

Every suggestion:
1. Will cause more problems elsewhere.
2. Has been tried before and failed.
3. Is a stopgap measure which does not get at the "real problem."
4. Can be implemented only if more space is provided.

Every problem can be described as:
1. Someone else's.
2. Originating outside of the department.
3. A result of lack of funds or people.
4. A problem which only more space will solve.

● ● ● ● ●

Life is a grindstone. Whether it polishes us or reduces us to dust depends on what we are made of.

● ● ● ● ●

The man who can smile when things go wrong has thought of someone to blame it on.

● ● ● ● ●